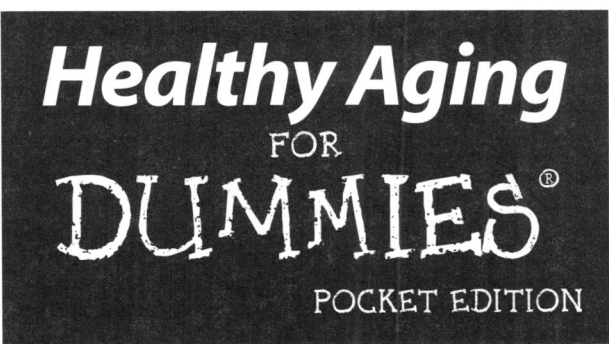

Healthy Aging
FOR
DUMMIES®
POCKET EDITION

by Brent Agin and Sharon Perkins

AF208014

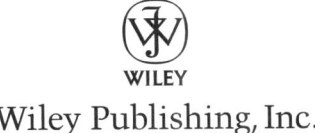

WILEY

Wiley Publishing, Inc.

Healthy Aging For Dummies,® Pocket Edition
Published by
Wiley Publishing, Inc.
111 River Street
Hoboken, NJ 07030-5774
www.wiley.com

Copyright © 2009 by Wiley Publishing, Inc., Indianapolis, Indiana

Published by Wiley Publishing, Inc., Indianapolis, Indiana

Published simultaneously in Canada

No part of this publication may be reproduced, stored in a retrieval system or transmitted in any form or by any means, electronic, mechanical, photocopying, recording, scanning or otherwise, except as permitted under Sections 107 or 108 of the 1976 United States Copyright Act, without either the prior written permission of the Publisher, or authorization through payment of the appropriate per-copy fee to the Copyright Clearance Center, 222 Rosewood Drive, Danvers, MA 01923, (978) 750-8400, fax (978) 646-8600. Requests to the Publisher for permission should be addressed to the Legal Department, Wiley Publishing, Inc., 10475 Crosspoint Blvd., Indianapolis, IN 46256, (317) 572-3447, fax (317) 572-4355, or online at http://www.wiley.com/go/permissions.

Trademarks: Wiley, the Wiley Publishing logo, For Dummies, the Dummies Man logo, A Reference for the Rest of Us!, The Dummies Way, Dummies Daily, The Fun and Easy Way, Dummies.com, and related trade dress are trademarks or registered trademarks of John Wiley & Sons, Inc. and/or its affiliates in the United States and other countries, and may not be used without written permission. All other trademarks are the property of their respective owners. Wiley Publishing, Inc., is not associated with any product or vendor mentioned in this book.

<u>LIMIT OF LIABILITY/DISCLAIMER OF WARRANTY</u>: THE PUBLISHER AND THE AUTHOR MAKE NO REPRESENTATIONS OR WARRANTIES WITH RESPECT TO THE ACCURACY OR COMPLETENESS OF THE CONTENTS OF THIS WORK AND SPECIFICALLY DISCLAIM ALL WARRANTIES, INCLUDING WITHOUT LIMITATION WARRANTIES OF FITNESS FOR A PARTICULAR PURPOSE. NO WARRANTY MAY BE CREATED OR EXTENDED BY SALES OR PROMOTIONAL MATERIALS. THE ADVICE AND STRATEGIES CONTAINED HEREIN MAY NOT BE SUITABLE FOR EVERY SITUATION. THIS WORK IS SOLD WITH THE UNDERSTANDING THAT THE PUBLISHER IS NOT ENGAGED IN RENDERING LEGAL, ACCOUNTING, OR OTHER PROFESSIONAL SERVICES. IF PROFESSIONAL ASSISTANCE IS REQUIRED, THE SERVICES OF A COMPETENT PROFESSIONAL PERSON SHOULD BE SOUGHT. NEITHER THE PUBLISHER NOR THE AUTHOR SHALL BE LIABLE FOR DAMAGES ARISING HEREFROM. THE FACT THAT AN ORGANIZATION OR WEBSITE IS REFERRED TO IN THIS WORK AS A CITATION AND/OR A POTENTIAL SOURCE OF FURTHER INFORMATION DOES NOT MEAN THAT THE AUTHOR OR THE PUBLISHER ENDORSES THE INFORMATION THE ORGANIZATION OR WEBSITE MAY PROVIDE OR RECOMMENDATIONS IT MAY MAKE. FURTHER, READERS SHOULD BE AWARE THAT INTERNET WEBSITES LISTED IN THIS WORK MAY HAVE CHANGED OR DISAPPEARED BETWEEN WHEN THIS WORK WAS WRITTEN AND WHEN IT IS READ.

For general information on our other products and services, please contact our Customer Care Department within the U.S. at 800-762-2974, outside the U.S. at 317-572-3993, or fax 317-572-4002.

For technical support, please visit www.wiley.com/techsupport.

Wiley also publishes its books in a variety of electronic formats. Some content that appears in print may not be available in electronic books.

ISBN: 978-0-470-41426-2

Manufactured in the United States of America

10 9 8 7 6 5 4 3 2 1

Table of Contents

Introduction

● ●

*I*f you're like many folks today, you realize that not only are people living longer than they used to, but also some of those people are living amazingly well while looking great. What's their secret to living such an independent, active, and radiant lifestyle? The answer lies in their healthy lifestyle. The goal of *Healthy Aging For Dummies,* Pocket Edition, is to educate you on the healthy choices you can make that reward you with a healthier, longer, happier life. Here are a few keys to success:

- ✔ **Prevention:** By arming yourself with solid knowledge and making changes to your current lifestyle, you won't necessarily live longer (although you may), but you will live a better *quality* of life.

- ✔ **Moderation:** Easy does it and in small doses. Making small but significant changes in your life can make a difference over time.

- ✔ **Timing:** Start now! Whether you are 20-something or 70-something, you are the CEO of your body, and it's up to you to manage it.

- ✔ **Practice:** Incorporating new routines in place of old habits takes some getting used to. But in time and with consistent practice, these lifestyle changes can become second nature.

It's never too early or too late to start taking care of your body. The sooner you treat your body as if it's the only one you're going to get, the sooner you're on your way to healthy aging.

Icons Used in This Book

This book uses icons — small graphics or images in the margins — to mark certain paragraphs of information that you may find useful. Here's the rundown of the helpful icons we use in this book.

When you see this icon, you'll find a helpful hint about doing something to help you age gracefully.

This icon denotes critical information that you need to take away with you. Be sure to read it.

The Warning icon cautions you against something that's potentially harmful. Be sure to read and heed the information with these icons.

Where to Go from Here

You've got your copy of *Healthy Aging For Dummies, Pocket Edition* — now what? This minibook is a reference, so if you want to know more about improving memory, head to Chapter 4. Or if you're interested in finding out more about macronutrients, flip to Chapter 3. Or heck, start with Chapter 1 and read the chapters in order . . . you rebel. If you want even more advice about healthy aging, from taking care of your skin to decreasing stress, check out the full-size version of *Healthy Aging For Dummies* — simply head to your local book seller or go to www.dummies.com.

Chapter 1
The Fountain of Youth, at Your Fingertips

* *

In This Chapter

▶ Understanding the current life expectancy

▶ Uncovering proven methods to combat aging

▶ Looking at the staggering numbers of preventable deaths

* *

*O*ver the years, thousands of people have searched for the elusive Fountain of Youth, and although some have claimed to have found it, for most, it remains a hidden treasure. Great strides have been made in uncovering the secrets to aging healthfully and lengthening the lifespan, but there's still progress to be made. As much as you may wish otherwise, most people know there's no magic pill for good health and longevity. It takes commitment, work, and sometimes even denial of self — giving up poor eating habits, a couch potato lifestyle, and the stressful schedules so many are addicted to — to stay healthy as you get older. You may be taking care of the externals but skipping over the basics of good health, which are also the basics of aging well.

You can't skip over the basics so easily, though. Balance is a big key in life, and healthy aging is no different. Skipping over essential healthcare is like ignoring routine maintenance on your car — the end result can be costly and dangerous.

Healthy aging is a current hot topic, and you can thank the baby boomer generation — the oldest of these people are now heading into their 60s — for today's emphasis on youthful, healthy aging. In this chapter, we discuss why people are living longer and better today than in previous generations, what impacted life expectancy a century ago, and what impacts our health and longevity today.

The Basics of Pro-Aging: The Best Actions You Can Take

You can't prevent the passage of time, but when you're *proactive* about your life choices, you can control some of the risk factors in your life associated with illness and disease.

You may not realize just how much control you have over how long you live — and we don't necessarily mean that in a good way. Seemingly casual choices you make every day may have the most profound impact on your health. In fact, it's estimated that if everyone in the United States led a healthy lifestyle, more than 50 percent of the cases of cardiovascular disease and diabetes could be avoided, and more than 50 percent of all cases of cancer prevented.

 The following tips show you how to avoid the most damaging and preventable threats to your health and aging:

✔ **Don't smoke — and if you already do, stop.**
Really. Smoking increases the risks for the top
three killers: heart disease, cancer, and cardiovascular ailments, including strokes. It also damages
your lungs and other parts of your respiratory
system. At least 60 chemicals in cigarette smoke
cause cancer, and as a cigarette burns, it produces
the poisons carbon monoxide, ammonia,
formaldehyde, arsenic, and cyanide.

✔ **Limit alcohol consumption.** If you drink alcohol,
no more than two drinks a day are safe for men,
and one or fewer drinks a day for women. (A stan-
dard drink is one 12-ounce bottle of beer or wine
cooler, one 5-ounce glass of wine, or 1.5 ounces of
80-proof distilled spirits.) Women are more likely
to have liver damage from drinking two or more
drinks a day than men are, so it's especially
important for women to keep alcohol consumption to one or fewer drinks a day.

Alcohol is a depressant and can exacerbate
the symptoms of depression and other mental
disturbances.

✔ **Maintain a healthy, balanced diet.** We can't over-
state the importance of a balanced and healthy diet
as you age. A poor diet can lead to an increased
risk of many health problems, including osteoporosis, heart disease, and impaired memory. Eating
well, on the other hand, makes you feel and look
better, keeps your body functioning optimally,
wards off colds and sickness, and contributes to
lowering blood pressure and cholesterol levels,
which in turn helps protect you against heart disease and stroke.

- ✔ **Exercise regularly.** Over time, a sedentary lifestyle can lead to obesity, a preventable yet dangerous epidemic that poses a threat to people's longevity. And it's on the rise. As you age, regular exercise should be a cornerstone of healthy living. As your body slows down, you may be tempted to skip the exercise because it's harder to do, you feel challenged physically, or you accept that being less active is part of normal aging. Don't fall prey to this thinking!

- ✔ **Manage your stress and develop healthy coping mechanisms.** Stress causes the release of the hormones cortisol, norepinephrine, and epinephrine, which under acute stress have a protective effect on the body. But *chronic* stress allows hormones to hang around longer than usual and cause the formation of free radicals

- ✔ **Get enough sleep regularly.** You need sleep, both psychologically and physiologically. The body uses this time for healing and growth, and your body produces many hormones essential for proper functioning during the deepest sleep stages. Sleep irregularity can have a direct impact on some disorders, such as epilepsy and migraines, and has been associated with diseases, such as cardiovascular disease, clinical depression, diabetes, and other serious conditions.

- ✔ **Visit your doctor for the recommended screening tests for your age.** Several important tests can help protect against cancer, heart disease, stroke, diabetes, and osteoporosis. Some of these tests find diseases early, when they're most treatable, while others can actually help keep a disease from developing in the first place.

If Staying Young and Healthy Is So Easy, Why Isn't Everyone Doing It?

There's nothing terribly complicated about living a healthy, life-prolonging lifestyle. So why are more people falling prey to partially preventable diseases every year? In this section, we explore what we think are the biggest reasons behind the staggering numbers of preventable death.

Short-sighted thinking

We're going to let you in on a little secret, everyone is mortal. Despite this being common knowledge, few people think about the inevitability of their own death and the things they can do to prevent it from happening prematurely. If they did, there would be far fewer accidents of every type, no one would ever break their hip falling off a ladder they shouldn't have been on in the first place, and cigarette sales would plummet.

The idea that death can be postponed leads to thinking that "tomorrow" is a good time to start a dietary overhaul, an ambitious new exercise regimen, and, of course, tomorrow is the best time to quit smoking and drinking. For many people, tomorrow is also a good time to finally call and set up the routine physical or breast exam they've been avoiding for the past five years.

 We're not advocating that you get out the sackcloth and ashes and carry a sign that states "The End is Near," but a little realism can go a long way toward a new way of living that can literally save lives — at least for a few more years.

Confusing what feels good with what is good

Making healthy food choices can have a major impact on health and aging. Most people know some of the fundamental eating habits that should be avoided such as eating fried foods and high sugar content snacks. Those same people also know that fruits and vegetables are good for you. Then why are so many people unable to make the decision to eat the way they know they should?

Could it be that some people's inability to stop eating poorly is an addiction, similar to addictions to tobacco and alcohol? More likely, it's the cavalier attitude many people have about their health that keeps them eating poorly, until they're slapped in the face with the reality of poor health. You may have heard the saying "cancer is the cure for smoking." Well, you would think diabetes and heart disease would be the cure for obesity . . . but sadly, they often aren't. This battle is never ending in the medical profession. Moving to healthy eating habits is difficult. Eating what's good for you just doesn't feel as good as eating what's bad for you, in many cases. It's not that you can't ever eat a fast food meal again — you can. You can't, however, eat fast food or packaged food all or even most of the time and stay healthy.

The desire for a quick (and easy) fix

Given a choice, most people will take the quick fix over hard work every time. Lose 25 pounds in a week, guaranteed? Sign me up! Quit smoking overnight? Here's my money! Build a beautiful body in only two minutes a day — and you don't even have to stand up? That's for me!

It's human nature to want something for nothing, but when it comes to living longer, you have to put in the time and effort — hours in the gym, self-control in the grocery store, and discipline in your lifestyle choices. And make no mistake, it takes time and effort to eat healthier foods, exercise, and maintain a focused, balanced low-stress lifestyle. You have to give up things — horribly unhealthy foods that taste so wonderful as well as time you feel short on anyway — to get yourself in a positive aging routine.

Modifying Your Lifestyle: The One True Source of Hope

Wading through the mire of information, articles, products, and research on aging is enough to leave you feeling conflicted and confused. Medicine is starting to center on the behavioral modification that effectively helps people practice healthy lifestyles. So familiarize yourself with the truth — which we provide for you in the pages of this book — and resolve to let it guide your decisions.

In the end, living a healthier lifestyle is nine-tenths attitude change and one-tenth real effort. If you change your attitude about food, eating healthy will no longer seem like a punishment. Changing your exercise attitude makes exercise a pleasure rather than a pain. Getting rest is the energy for tomorrow. This type of attitude pushes you forward through the rest of this book and educates you further about the dangers and rewards of better lifestyles and healthier aging. And we're happy to take the first leg of your journey to healthful living and aging with you.

Chapter 2
Evaluating Your Health and Setting Goals

. . . .

In This Chapter

▶ Getting the facts on your medical history

▶ Keeping those appointments and test dates

▶ Setting personal goals for a healthier you

. . . .

*P*eople used to go to the doctor only when they were sick or had broken a bone. And plenty of people still cower or scoff at the idea of visiting the doctor when they're ill, let alone getting a checkup if they're feeling just dandy — you know, the *if it ain't broke, don't fix it!* rule. Well, we don't happen to prescribe to that philosophy as a recipe for longevity or even good health.

In this chapter, we discuss the general measures you can implement to prevent the most threatening illnesses and diseases today. Because your body doesn't come with an owner's manual to tell you when it's time for a tuneup, we tell you what to look for, what age to start looking, and what tests or screenings to schedule with your healthcare provider. Then we help you put your goals down on paper and devise a plan that will keep you from giving up when the going gets tough.

Investigating Your Family History

Knowing your family history can give you a blueprint of potential health landmines in your genetic makeup. Your doctor needs to know about any family history of illness, such as cardiovascular disease, cancer, and so on, because it can change prevention, testing, and treatments due to certain familial links.

When compiling a family health history, start with your immediate family — brothers, sisters, mom, and dad — and then move on to extended family. You can start by asking questions of your parents, such as:

- **How long did your parents live and what did they die of?** You may not get a straight answer on the cause of your grandparents' deaths, because often cause of death wasn't accurately recorded a generation or so ago. Even deaths recorded as accidents may not be accurate; a "car accident" may have been caused by a sudden heart attack.

- **Did they have any health problems?** Try to get specifics; "bad blood" could be anything from anemia to syphilis! Some of the more common conditions with genetic links are heart disease, cancer, addiction, and diabetes.

- **What do you remember about them?** They may remember that grandma was blind and had only one leg without making the connection that these conditions may have been caused by diabetes.

✔ **Do you have any pictures of relatives?** One
  look at a series of pictures of great grandma and
  grandma at different ages can make it evident that
  osteoporosis runs in the family — they kept getting shorter!

✔ **Did any diseases or defects "run in the family"?**
  Expect some waffling on the answer if mental conditions or birth defects were common in the
  family. Explain your need to know as a desire to
  understand your family medical history rather
  than pure nosiness.

✔ **What about your brothers and sisters and their
  families?** Make sure that you're recording health
  issues only from blood relatives, not their spouses
  or their in-laws.

After you gather enough data to make up a
cohesive family history, write it all down. The
U.S. Surgeon General considers your family
history recording important enough to have
devised a personalized form that you can use
to record pertinent info; you can find it at
`www.familyhistory.hhs.gov`.

Visiting the Doc

Some people would rather have a tax audit than go to
the doctor. The main reason? Fear — and fear of the
unknown only perpetuates the problem. But taking
your body to the doctor for regular checkups is an
important part of living long and well. To make sure
that you cover your bases, we devote this section to
those appointments.

Having regular checkups: What should happen

As long as you're feeling okay, you probably don't think about getting a physical exam — not good for two reasons:

✔ Prevention is the key to reducing your risks of developing disease and illness, so if you don't take advantage of your doctor's insight regarding your risks, you're missing out on a key component of aging healthfully.

✔ When you do visit the doctor regularly, you can immediately address any health concerns the doctor may find; if you don't, you may not know about those health concerns soon enough to combat them before they take their toll on your body.

 For folks ages 40 and older, we highly recommend health examinations every one to two years. (Younger adults don't need the exam this often — every three to five years is good.)

During the annual exam, your doctor performs the assessments in the following sections.

Discussing current medical complaints

The first part of the exam is an opportunity to discuss your current medical situation so that it can be further evaluated throughout the rest of the examination.

The review of your body systems is a way for the doctor to assess your overall health quickly (and sufficiently). You'll be asked a number of questions to gather information to direct the diagnosis, treatment, and prevention.

Reviewing past medical information

At this stage of the examination your doctor will want to go over past medical information that may pertain to your current medical complaints. This is a good point to whip out your comprehensive family history to help your doctor assess for possible inherited problems and tendencies.

Checking your vitals

Vital signs are a group of measured tests that help give a quick assessment of a patient's basic bodily function. These functions include blood pressure, pulse, respirations, and temperature. A few other measurements can be thrown into this mix, including height, weight, pulse oximetry (a noninvasive measure of the oxygenation in your blood), and pain. Sometimes this step happens at the beginning of your appointment, and sometimes it happens after you go over all the history.

At last, undergoing the physical exam

Sooner or later, you have to put on that skimpy gown and sit on the crinkly-paper-covered exam table to get checked out. Your doctor examines you from head to toe, checking most of your orifices, squeezing muscles, and pointing out any abnormalities to discuss and possibly test further:

- ✔ **General appearance:** You'd be surprised what you can assess just looking at someone. Mobility, mood, skin color, and hygiene can all be evaluated within a minute or two of general conversation.

✔ **Skin:** Doctors check the skin for any suspicious rashes or moles.

✔ **Head, ears, eyes, neck, throat (HEENT):** Examination of the head basically consists of checking the ears, mouth, and nose. Evaluating the visual fields and papillary reaction, and testing with an eye chart are included in an eye exam. To examine your throat, a doctor checks for neck stiffness, thyroid enlargement, and lymph node swelling.

✔ **Cardiovascular:** The doctor checks your vital signs by listening to the heart for any abnormal rhythm or sounds, checking for any swelling of the extremities or varicose veins, and listening to the carotid arteries of the neck for any signs of blockage.

✔ **Respiratory:** After checking the respiratory rate, your doctor listens to the lungs for any wheezing, lack of breath sounds, or other sounds suggestive of disease.

✔ **Gastrointestinal:** Your doctor listens for bowel sounds, and presses on the abdomen looking for pain, masses, hernias, or abdominal distention.

✔ **Genitourinary and rectal:** For men this includes evaluation of the penis and scrotum, including evaluating the testicles for any masses. The female exam is discussed in the next list (see the Pap smear bullet). Patients start getting rectal exams at age 40 unless otherwise needed; doctors use this exam to check for hemorrhoids and to evaluate the prostate for any enlargement or masses.

✔ **Musculoskeletal:** Your doctor evaluates range of motion and muscle strength, and checks the spine for straightness and any tenderness. Your doctor also listens for *crepitus,* a creaking sound, when your joints are moved.

✔ **Extremities:** Your doctor evaluates your extremities for swelling and any abnormalities in the muscles. He feels the pulses in the knee and foot, and looks for any enlarged lymph nodes in the groin.

✔ **Neurological:** The doc checks reflexes of the knees, feet, and elbow by tapping them with a small hammer. Your doctor may check your gait by watching you walk, and then check your feet and hands for sensory defects.

Other tests are often done at the time of routine examinations and are just as important, but not all these tests are done at every annual examination. A few of these important tests are done at different set times or when other circumstances arise. Here are a few tests to expect at some point, whether annually or not:

✔ **Pap smear:** From the time you become sexually active or turn 18 (whichever comes first), you should have a yearly Pap smear until age 30. After age 30, women have Pap smears every three years after three yearly negative tests in a row. Pap smears may be discontinued after age 65 if previous screenings (a minimum of three negative Pap tests in the last ten years) are normal and documented.

✔ **Clinical breast exams and mammograms:** Because breast care is one of the most important aspects of women's healthcare, clinical breast exams should begin at age 20. Women age 40 and older should have a mammogram every year.

✔ **Prostate cancer screening:** Prostate cancer is the second leading cause of cancer deaths among men. Each year, men age 40 and older should have both of the following tests:

- **A prostate specific antigen (PSA) screening test.** The PSA is a simple blood test that in some cases can detect cancer in the prostate before signs and symptoms are present. The only problem is that it isn't always accurate. Therefore, the PSA shouldn't be used as a diagnostic tool, but it can be helpful to monitor the treatment of prostate cancer.

- **A digital rectal exam.** This test is done to assess the size of the prostate and palpate for any other abnormalities, such as pain or masses.

Less frequent exams

Some tests need to be done only when you reach a certain age, have certain risk factors, or are having problems in a particular area. The following list describes some of the tests that fall into this category:

✔ **Cholesterol screening:** Every five years, all adults should have a *lipid profile,* a cholesterol test done after you've had nothing to eat or drink for 12 hours (called a "fasting" test) that assesses all the components of cholesterol: total, HDL or good cholesterol, LDL or bad cholesterol, and triglycerides.

✔ **Eye exam:** Plan to have an eye examination at least once from age 18 to 29, at least twice from age 30 to 39, every two to four years from age 40 to 64, and every one to two years thereafter.

- ✔ **Fasting blood sugar screening:** Fasting blood sugar should be measured every three years, starting at age 45, to screen for *diabetes mellitus,* one of the most commonly undiagnosed diseases.

- ✔ **Colorectal cancer screening:** A complete colonoscopy and examination of the intestines are done using a flexible lighted scope while you're under mild sedation. People age 50 and older should have this test done every ten years — and more frequently if you have a family history of colon cancer or a previous abnormal colonoscopy.

- ✔ **Bone-mineral density exam:** Women age 65 and older should have a bone mineral density measurement at least once to check for *osteoporosis,* a disease in which bones become fragile and more likely to break.

- ✔ **Hearing test:** Adults over the age of 64 should have at least one hearing assessment. Your health-care provider will ask about your hearing, and if you're having difficulty or noticing small changes, he will probably recommend a hearing test. Proper treatment, including cleaning or treating infections, can greatly improve your ability to hear.

Determining Your Goals and Putting Them on Paper

To achieve goals, you need plans. But the simpler the plan, and the less disruption it causes to your daily life, the more likely you are to stick to it. Think of your body as a machine that needs certain maintenance. Plan on the regular, routine maintenance and if any signs of breakdown appear, get to the doctor sooner rather than later to prevent any worsening of the situation. The body is complex and therefore is somewhat unpredictable, so accept that you have to adapt to changes and make adjustments to keep the body aging well.

Developing your goals

When determining and implementing your goals, follow a few guidelines to make them effective:

✔ **Develop your goals as clearly as possible.** Each goal should be defined as a specific task that's action oriented so that you can actually do something to accomplish it. Having a goal of "losing weight" isn't as clear as "losing five pounds a month by cutting out afternoon and after dinner snacks and walking two miles a day." The second goal has specific, action oriented tasks for you to work on.

✔ **Make sure that your goals are measurable.** With goals, if you can't measure them, how do you know whether you've accomplished them? The difference between a goal and a wish is as simple as these two statements:

- I want to lose weight.
- I want to lose 25 pounds.

The second statement is actually a goal.

✔ **Set firm but realistic deadlines.** There isn't much point of having a goal if you never set a time frame to reach it.

✔ **Own your goals.** Many people don't stick to their goals because they don't really take ownership of them. Your goals must be a burning desire for *you* — not for someone else. Whether your goal is going to the gym four days a week, eating healthy food to lose weight and maintain it, choosing a positive attitude over a negative one, or protecting your skin from sun damage — every goal has obstacles. Choose goals that you're passionate about. You're much more likely to achieve them.

Recording your goals

Plenty of research supports the effective correlation between writing down your goals and achieving them. Here's why we also believe in the power of this process:

- ✔ Writing down your goals forces you to organize your thinking.

- ✔ Thinking about what you must do to accomplish your goals helps you to plan your tasks more thoughtfully.

- ✔ A well-written plan provides the ability to review it for flaws as well as to identify strengths and weaknesses.

- ✔ A written plan allows you to focus on just a few key objectives.

- ✔ Writing your plan ahead of time instead of flying by the seat of your pants saves time, energy, confusion, and mistakes.

Finding support

Unless you're a Lone Ranger type (and even he had a sidekick!), you're likely to find lifestyle changes like dieting, quitting smoking, and starting an exercise program much easier if you have company along the way. A good friend or a whole support group of people can encourage you, help you get back on track when you waver, and cheer you on when you succeed. Plus, a little healthy competition may spur you all on to success. The beauty is that you can find people who specialize in helping you achieve your goals if you find it hard to go it alone.

Finding support for specific goals can be simple. Want to quit smoking? Find a friend or relative to team up with, or join a group like Nicotine Anonymous, a spinoff organization of Alcoholics Anonymous. Diet plans? You can find dozens, both online and live, to choose from. Not interested in baring your problems in public? Look for the hundreds, if not thousands, of online support groups for every type of issue under the sun, including support for specific diet plans and forums that discuss exercise videos made by different groups or individuals.

Just making your goal known to someone else — even if it's just your mom or best friend — increases the likelihood that you'll stick with it. Want to make the stakes higher? Organize a group where each person contributes a monetary amount and the person closest to his or her goal after a set time wins the pot. Or make your own personal reward system; put money toward something you really want and then hand the money to someone else to "keep" for you until you reach your goal.

"Going it alone" can be successful, but it can be a lonely road. Team up with friends or make some new ones and the journey toward your goals will seem much shorter — and a lot more fun, too.

Chapter 3
You Are What You Eat:
Nutrition 101

In This Chapter

▶ Knowing the importance of nutrition as you age

▶ Checking out foods that are good for your body

▶ Living a healthy life and making healthy habits

▶ Reading labels on your food

he phrase "Garbage in, garbage out" is just as true for your body as it is for your computer. If your diet lacks nutrients, or if you eat too much or too little, the results show up as health problems and feeling ill, especially as you age.

In this chapter, we look at the importance of good nutrition (and we define it) and how your body's nutritional needs may change as you age.

The Importance of Nutrients — and Why You Should Care

Most everything you put in your mouth has some nutrients, but some foods have more *macronutrients* — nutrients that your body uses in larger amounts, which comprise proteins, carbs, and fats — and micronutrients — nutrients that your body requires in smaller amounts, such as vitamins and minerals — than others. In addition, some foods have additional properties that promote extra health benefits and help boost your immune system, which weakens as you age. These additional components may include the following:

- **Antioxidants:** These compounds help fight free radicals that result from oxidation. *Oxidation* is the loss of electrons in atoms; free radicals can damage cells and cause disease or deterioration in your body. Oxidation appears to increase as you age, making antioxidants a valuable player on the anti-aging field.

  Foods that contain vitamins A, C, and E, beta carotene, selenium, and lycopene (found in tomatoes) are rich with antioxidants. Most brightly colored fruits and vegetables contain essential antioxidants too, which are more beneficial when consumed in food than taken in supplement form. Antioxidants also help keep your immune system strong.

- **Bioflavanoids:** Bioflavanoids are the brightly colored pigments found in fruits, red wine, and vegetables; they're a class of antioxidants (see preceding bullet) necessary for vitamin C absorption. They also strengthen blood vessels and have anti-inflammatory properties.

- **Omega-3 and -6 fatty acids:** These essential oils are found in some fish, meats, eggs, walnuts, corn, safflower, and oils such as canola and flaxseed. Studies show that they may protect against heart disease by lowering triglyceride blood levels as well as possibly decreasing rheumatoid arthritis, depression, macular degeneration, and asthma. These fatty acids are best utilized by the body when obtained from food instead of supplements.

✔ **Phyoestrols:** Phyoestrols are found in plants; they work to lower LDL (low density lipoproteins, the "bad" cholesterol) blood levels. There are two types of phyoestrols: sterols and stanols. Both are found in fruits, legumes, nuts, seeds, vegetables, and vegetable oils. Some food products are fortified by phyesterols. These foods include orange juice, some cereals, salad dressing, and lowfat milk.

✔ **Probiotics:** Probiotics are living microorganisms that positively benefit you. They improve the health and functioning of your gastrointestinal tract (GI) and may help boost your immune system. Probiotics such as bacteria and yeast help balance the flora (microorganisms) found in your intestinal tract, killing off the bad bacteria and allowing the good bacteria to flourish.

✔ **Prebiotics:** Prebiotics are found in whole grains, bananas, honey, onions, artichokes, and fortified food products. They also help balance flora in the GI tract and may aid in calcium absorption.

How Nutritional Needs Change As You Age

The aging process affects the body's absorption of many micronutrients. You need to take in more nutrients to absorb the same amount, or you may become deficient in that vitamin or mineral.

As you age, focus on increasing the levels of the following nutrients:

✔ **Calcium:** Hormonal changes may decrease calcium absorption as it increases loss of calcium through the kidneys. In addition, you may become *lactose intolerant* (lose some of your ability to digest lactose, the sugar in milk). Because of this condition, some people decrease their intake of dairy products, which are good sources of calcium. But you still need to get the calcium from somewhere. Most people don't eat enough dairy products or veggies to get adequate calcium from their diet and should consider supplementation. The amount of calcium can vary with age or medical conditions, but in general adults should have about 1,000 mg a day, and if you're over the age of 50 increase the dose to 1,200 mg daily.

✔ **Iron:** Iron is necessary to carry oxygen to your cells, but it's difficult to get all you need because most foods contain only a little iron. The best source of iron is in red meat, but you can also get iron from poultry, fish, whole grain or enriched breads and cereals, dry beans, and some fruits and vegetables. Women over age 50 should get 50 mg of iron a day where as men only need 10 mg.

 Vitamin C helps you absorb more iron from foods, so be sure you include foods with vitamin C (such as citrus fruits, greens, and tomatoes) in the same meal as foods with iron.

 Taking too many iron supplements can be lethal. Talk to your doctor before taking iron supplements.

Picking the Right Macronutrients (Protein, Carbs, and Fats)

The changes in recommendations on what type of macronutrients are best for you from year to year may have you feeling a bit like Alice in Wonderland — which foods make you healthy, which ones make you sick?

In the next section, we help you figure out how to pick the best macronutrients out of the bewildering number of choices available.

Consuming complete proteins, no matter your lifestyle

Protein is a dietary essential, even for vegans who don't eat animal protein in any way, shape, or form. Proteins are made up of tissue building blocks called *amino acids,* and proteins that contain all the *essential amino acids* (amino acids that the body can't make and therefore must be obtained in foods) are called "complete." Animal protein is a good example of a complete protein, while the proteins found in grains, nuts, and vegetables are incomplete, and you must carefully balance them to obtain all the essential amino acids in your diet.

Although protein isn't a high source of energy, your body uses proteins to grow and to build hormones, antibodies, and the enzymes that regulate the chemical reactions within the body. Proteins are essential for healthy aging because they maintain healthy tissues and sustain growth. Because protein can't be stored in the body, you need a new supply every day to keep tissues from breaking down.

Getting just enough

The U.S. Department of Agriculture (USDA) says that to be healthy, 20 percent of your total daily calories should come from protein. So if your optimal daily caloric intake is 1,800 calories, 360 of them should be in the form of protein.

Considering the source

Red meat is a good source of complete protein, but some red meat also contains a large amount of saturated fat, which can raise your cholesterol levels and contribute to heart disease. So poultry and fish, which contain less saturated fat, provide a better source of protein. And if you're vegetarian, you don't have to worry about the high levels of saturated fats in meat — dry beans and nuts are excellent sources of protein. Most servings of protein supply around 24 grams of protein.

 Your protein needs depend on your activity level, age, and if you're dieting. Use the following equation to calculate your protein needs:

Weight x 0.6 grams of protein per pound

For example: 170 pounds $\times$ 0.6 = 102 grams of protein per day. Remember that this formula is an approximation. Check with your doctor, too.

You can break down your protein choices like this:

✔ **Complete proteins:** These contain all essential amino acids. Examples include the following:

  • **Beef:** Lean beef contains less than 10 percent fat, but be careful — this doesn't apply to ground beef, which, in some states, doesn't even have to display the exact fat content on the label. Mix ground turkey with regular ground beef to cut the fat.

- **Poultry (chicken, turkey, and duck):** The white meat in poultry is high in protein, low in fat, and low in cholesterol. Remember to remove the skin (that's where most of the fat is) and stick to white meat, which has less fat than dark meat. Poultry contains about 0.5 grams of saturated fat and delivers a walloping 30 plus grams of protein per serving.

- **Fish:** Some fish is very low in saturated fats; most types of fish have less than 1 gram of saturated fat per serving. A few have 2 grams — salmon and tuna among them. Fish is a good source of protein as long as you don't fry it in saturated fat. Fish is also a good source of omega-3 fatty acids. The fish that's best for these fatty acids include salmon, tuna, trout, mackerel, and whitefish. Fish contains around 20 grams of protein per serving.

- **Pork:** Pork has about the same amount of saturated fat (2 grams per serving) as lean beef, even when you trim the fat before eating. Although the pork industry is promoting it as the "other white meat," pork is higher in saturated fat than poultry and shouldn't be a nightly dinner choice. Pork has around 25 grams of protein per serving.

- **Lamb:** Lamb is also high in fat compared to poultry; in fact, it's slightly higher (3 grams per serving) than pork in saturated fat.

- **Eggs:** Eggs contain about 6.25 grams of protein and are only 75 calories. The egg white is only 17 calories. They have 3.5 grams of saturated fat, which is mostly contained in the yolk, but the yolk contains most of the amino acids and 40 percent of the protein.

✔ **Incomplete proteins:** These don't contain all essential amino acids. Incomplete proteins include

- **Dry beans:** Dry beans and lentils are excellent sources of protein, although you may not think of them as such. Beans contain around 7 grams of protein and lentils about 9 grams protein per half cup and less than one gram of saturated fat. To obtain all the essential amino acids, you need to combine them with other sources of protein that contain the rest of the essential amino acids.

- **Nuts:** Nuts are a good source of protein, around 5 grams per serving, but are also high in saturated fats; a serving contains anywhere from 4 grams (almonds) to 16 grams (brazil nuts). Macadamia nuts are also high in saturated fats, about 12 grams per serving. Nuts are also an incomplete source of protein.

Choosing good carbs

Carbohydrates are an important part of your diet because they help supply the energy that your body needs to function. They are so important that the USDA recommends that half of your daily calorie intake should come from carbs. Carbohydrates fall into two categories:

> ✔ Simple, which contain refined sugars, with minimal fiber, vitamins, and minerals

> ✔ Complex, which contain more fiber, vitamins, and minerals

All carbohydrates are broken down and used for energy. The goal when choosing carbs is to chose complex carbs that increase energy storage at a slow, steady pace, to help control blood sugar levels. Sugars (simple carbs) are broken down most easily and cause a quick infusion of glucose (blood sugar) into your blood. This surge gives an immediate boost of energy, but it also causes blood sugar to drop rapidly and can leave you feeling weak.

Separating healthy carbs and unhealthy carbs: The glycemic index

Today, there's an increased emphasis on the glycemic index (GI) of foods. The glycemic index categorizes foods by how quickly they're broken down and enter the bloodstream and how high your blood sugar rises after eating them compared to pure glucose. Foods with a low glycemic index are considered most healthy. They're rated on a scale from 0-100, with the lower numbers being healthiest.

Sugars have a high glycemic index, while starches such as whole grains have a lower glycemic index and stabilize your blood sugar because they take longer to break down. (Fibers can't be broken down in the body and pass through unchanged.) So starches like whole grains and vegetables with a low glycemic index are your best choice for carbohydrates. Processed foods like white bread are stripped of much of the fiber, vitamins, and minerals, and they have a higher glycemic index, making less processed food like whole grain bread a much healthier choice.

Assessing a food's carbohydrate makeup: Glycemic load

Just to complicate things, carbohydrates are further categorized by their *glycemic load* (GL), which takes into consideration the amount of carbohydrates consumed. Two items might be similar on the GI but your blood sugars and insulin response are affected differently if you eat a greater amount of one than the other, which is the GL. You determine the glycemic load by taking the GI, dividing by 100, then multiplying by the carbohydrate count in the food. For example:

1. **A cup of cooked spaghetti has a GI of 42.**

   42 ÷ by 100 = .42.

2. **A cup of cooked spaghetti contains 38 carbs (subtract fiber, if any, from the total carb count since it isn't digested).**

   .42 × 38 = 16. So 16 is GL for a cup of cooked spaghetti.

 Anything below 10 is considered low, anything over 20 is considered high.

Fighting off the bad fats and getting enough of the good ones

You may be conditioned to think of fat as something bad to eat, but you need "good" fat in your diet for your body to function properly. You need fat to help with absorption of fat soluble vitamins, to regulate cholesterol metabolism, and to keep your skin soft and healthy.

Eating fat doesn't make you fat. Excess body fat comes from consuming too many calories (of any kind) that aren't used as energy but are stored away in the body as fat reserves.

Fat is either saturated or unsaturated:

✔ Saturated fat can be included in your diet, but should be limited due to the risks of elevated cholesterol.

✔ Unsaturated fat is good for you, lowering your LDL and raising your HDL.

Gathering near the good fats

Most people don't realize that fat plays a necessary role in their diet. The important thing is to make sure you have the right balance of good and bad fats. Healthy fats such as polyunsaturated and monounsaturated fats are beneficial to your body, but they need to be consumed in moderation.

Experts don't always agree on exactly what percentage of your daily calories should come from fat. According to the World Health Organization (WHO) people should restrict dietary fat intake to 30 percent of daily calories, and according to the USDA, you *need* 30 percent of your daily calories from fats. The American Heart Association suggests 20 to 30 percent, while some experts believe that people may only need as little as 10 percent of calories in the form of fat.

 You don't need to add a lot of extra fat to your diet; just make healthy food and cooking choices to get enough of the nutrients from the healthy fats you need.

Omega-3 fatty acids are one type of "good fat." There are many supplements that provide these fatty acids, because most people don't consume enough of the foods that contain omega-3s. Good sources of the omega-3 fatty acids are found in the following foods:

- ✔ Cold-water fish like mackerel, salmon, sardines, anchovies, and herring. The oils of wild-caught fish contain a significantly higher proportion of Omega-3 than the oils of farm-raised fish.

- ✔ Nuts, such as walnuts, Brazil nuts, and almonds along with pumpkin, sunflower, and flax seeds.

Saying no to the bad fats

Saturated fats and trans fats are bad for your health for the following reasons:

- ✔ **Saturated fats** are usually solid at room temperature, and they're a major dietary factor in raising cholesterol. The main sources of saturated fat in the typical American diet are foods from animals and some plants. These sources include whole milk, butter, cheese, ice cream, red meat and dark meat, milk chocolate, coconuts, coconut milk, and coconut oil.

- ✔ **Trans fats** should be avoided altogether because they can raise your total LDL (bad) cholesterol *and* lower HDL (good) cholesterol, putting you at risk for high blood pressure and heart disease. Examples of trans fat include most margarines, vegetable shortening, partially hydrogenated vegetable oil, deep-fried anything, many fast foods, and most commercially baked goods.

According to the USDA, no more than 10 percent of your daily calories should come from saturated fats. There's no official recommendation from the USDA for trans fats percentage, so we recommend that if you eat them at all, you share your 10-percent allotment between the two.

Reading Food Labels

Food labels have moved way outside the supermarket; everything from fast food to restaurant menus these days contain nutritional breakdowns of calorie count, percentages of protein, carbs and fat, calcium and iron recommended daily allowance (RDA) percentages, and much more in grams, milligrams, or percentages. There's no excuse today for not knowing what you're eating!

While food labels are a great source of info, and some-times even more than you want to know, they do have some caveats. For one thing, the percentages of RDA are based on a 2,000 calorie a day diet, with 60 percent of calories coming from carbohydrates, ten percent from protein, and thirty percent from fat, based on the average nutritional needs of a 170 pound man. If you're not a 170 pound man, but a 100 pound woman, the RDA percentage of, say, fat, contained in a food may not be accurate for you.

By law, all food labels contain the following information:

✔ **Serving size:** The most important thing to remember is that the serving size may not be the whole box, bag, or container. This fact may be obvious when you're looking at a 20 ounce bag of chips and not so obvious with a two-ounce bag.

✔ **Servings per container or package:** This information states the number of servings in the package. Don't forget — check this info *before* you start eating!

✔ **Calories and Calories from Fat:** The calorie content is important because excess intake can lead to weight gain. And the calories-from-fat number is crucial to help you limit fat intake, especially saturated and trans fats. Ideally the calories from fat should equal no more than 30 percent of the total number of calories in a serving.

✔ **% Daily Value:** This information compares the contents of the product to the RDA based on a 2,000-calorie diet. These numbers help you judge whether the food has enough or too much of the nutrients you need. For example, a box of macaroni and cheese (prepared) has 48 grams of carbohydrates, which is 16 percent of the RDA.

✔ **Total Fat, Carbohydrates, Protein, Cholesterol, Sodium:** This part of the label lists several important numbers. The label identifies the specific types of fat in the product (unsaturated, saturated, and trans fat) and their amounts. No more than 10 percent of your total 30 percent daily allowance of fat should come from saturated fats or trans fats. This label also helps if you're trying to track your carb and protein intake, your daily sodium intake, or if you're trying to cut down on cholesterol.

✔ **Vitamins and Minerals:** Percentages of RDA will also be listed on the food label, although it may be way too small for you to read without a magnifying glass!

Chapter 4
Maintaining a Healthy Body and a Sharp Mind

. . . .

In This Chapter

▶ Surveying body mass and the consequences of extra pounds

▶ Knowing your present health before setting future goals

▶ Getting on track with your personal plan

▶ Recognizing brain changes related to aging

▶ Training your brain to stay young

. . . .

*I*t's a sad story, but the vast majority of folks nowadays are on the fast track to fat like a runaway freight train in a summer blockbuster movie. The saddest part isn't so much the daily discomfort and inconvenience as it's the cumulative effects of lugging around those extra lipids. That added weight can actually take years off your life and possibly plague your days with illness and disease.

In this chapter we take you through the process of reaching your fitness goals even when they seem overwhelming. We also give you some tips on how to keep your brain functioning at maximum potential as you age.

Understanding Healthy Body Weight

Your ideal body weight is the eventual weight that your body adjusts to when you have a consistently healthy approach to eating and exercise. Your body wants to naturally maintain this weight based on your physiological makeup. It may take some time to determine this number if you have weight to lose or if you're underweight now.

 The most common method for determining your ideal weight is the *body mass index* (BMI), a mathematical calculation of a person's ideal mass (weight) based on his or her height and weight.

The BMI doesn't discriminate between muscle, fat, or bone. People who know that they're at their ideal weight based on their nutrition and other fat measurements can and should ignore the BMI; if you have a greater amount of muscle than most people, this generalized calculation isn't going to apply to you.

In general, however, a person's BMI score is a relatively good tool for people between the ages of 18 and 65.

Calculating body mass

Figuring out your body mass index sounds like an exercise in quantum physics, but don't despair; plenty of online tables do the work of calculating your BMI for you, given your height and weight. However, if you're the mathematical type who wants to check your figures against the tables, use the following formula:

Calculate BMI by dividing weight in pounds (lbs) by height in inches (in) squared, and multiplying by a conversion factor of 703.

Weight (lb) ÷ [height (in)]^2 × 703

Example: Weight = 170 lbs, Height = 6' (72")

Calculation: $[170 ÷ (72)^2] × 703 = 23.05$

Recognizing unhealthy body mass

By BMI standards, people with a body mass index of less than 18.5 are underweight, and those with a BMI of 20 to 25 are within range of their ideal body weight. For the most part, the higher the BMI, the higher the associated health risks. If your BMI goes over 25, you're creeping into the dreaded "overweight" category. Following is a breakdown of the categories of BMIs that are outside the ideal range:

- ✔ **Underweight:** A person with a body mass index (BMI) of 18.5 or less is considered underweight. Just as with being overweight, the BMI is a tool and having a low BMI may not mean that you're unhealthy. Often underweight individuals are perfectly healthy. If you experience any symptoms such as fatigue, thinning hair or nails, irregularity in periods (women), continuous weight loss, abdominal pains, or any other symptoms, see your doctor for further evaluation.

- ✔ **Overweight:** A person with a body mass index (BMI) of 25 to 29.9. Approximately 127 million adults (or 60.5 percent) in the U.S. are overweight. About 1 billion people in the world are overweight.

- ✔ **Obese:** A person with a BMI of 30 to 39.9. About 60 million adults (or 25 percent) in the U.S. are obese and 300 million obese adults exist worldwide. This number doesn't include children — one of the fastest growing obesity groups.

- ✔ **Morbidly obese:** A person 100 pounds over his normal weight or with a BMI of 40 or more. In the U.S., 9 million adults (or 5 percent) are morbidly obese. This group has a definite increase in obesity-related illness and mortality. The good news is that people in this BMI category *can* lose the weight, just like the people in the other weight categories. Get motivated and consult your physician to get a weight loss plan.

Assessing Your Current Level of Health

So, where do you begin? This section tells you how to get ready for the battle of the bulge — check in with your physician before checking in at the gym. We also look at what you need to know about your own health before you can tailor those workouts to be beneficial and safe. Finally, we cover your current weight and your goal weight to give you a good idea of the road ahead.

Evaluating your fitness level

Before beginning an exercise routine, ask yourself, "What's my baseline fitness level?" Translation: How active are you? Are you overweight? Do you exercise now? How many minutes a week do you exercise? Do you lift weights or do aerobic exercise? These questions give you, your doctor, and/or your personal trainer an idea of what your basic fitness level is.

The best personal fitness assessment comes from a personal trainer. Some gyms include the cost of an assessment as part of your membership, although others don't. You may also want to contact a local personal trainer specifically for this service.

An assessment can help you determine:

- The level of weights you should begin using
- How many days a week you should train
- How long you should train each workout day
- Which muscle groups require the most work

Getting the green light from your primary physician

Checking with a doctor before starting an exercise routine or weight-loss program is much more than just a legal disclaimer, so don't let this advice go in one ear and out the other. Some conditions and symptoms may require medical attention prior to jumping into exercise, just to make sure that your new exercise plan is right for you.

If you're not sure whether you need to see a doctor before starting a new or restarting an old exercise program, go through this health questionnaire. A "yes" answer to any of these questions means that you should consult a medical doctor first:

- Are you over the age of 40?
- Are you overweight?

- ✔ Do you smoke?

- ✔ Have you been sedentary for a long time?

- ✔ Are you starting an exercise program that involves more than walking or light weights?

- ✔ Has a doctor told you that you have a heart murmur?

- ✔ Has anyone in your family died of heart disease prior to the age of 55?

- ✔ Do you have a high risk of coronary heart disease or stroke?

- ✔ Do you have any medical conditions, such as high cholesterol, diabetes, high blood pressure, or kidney disease?

- ✔ Do your ankles swell?

- ✔ Have you experienced severe pain in your leg muscles while walking?

- ✔ Do you get short of breath more than usual when you're performing routine tasks?

- ✔ Have you fainted or do you have dizziness?

- ✔ Have you experienced any abnormal heartbeats or chest pain either at rest or when exerting yourself?

Custom-Designing Your Plan with Balance in Mind

The simple math is this: The cause of weight gain is eating more calories than you burn. Your body gains one pound for every 3,500 calories it doesn't use.

People who exercise daily throughout their lives maintain their ideal body weight more easily than those who don't. We can't stress this fact enough.

Creating a safe and effective exercise program

After a doctor clears you to exercise, and you have some physical assessments done, you should be able to compile a personalized exercise program to follow.

Covering the bases: The components of a complete routine

A common misconception for people who are just starting a routine is to focus only on cardio. But in that case, your body burns the energy stored in your muscles first and burns fat only as a last resort. (We know — it's a frustrating arrangement!) So, a body transformation occurs most efficiently by *simultaneously* gaining muscle through strength training and losing fat through aerobics and diet.

Keep these facts in mind as you build your personalized program:

- **Aerobic training:** Activities like walking, swimming, and biking are all good for the lungs and heart.

- **Strength training:** This is the only activity that slows muscle and bone loss while it promotes weight loss.

  Your body needs energy to sustain muscle mass because muscle cells are *metabolically demanding* (high-maintenance); for every pound of muscle you add, your body burns 30 to 50 more calories a day even at rest. How's that for a great bargain!

If you're just beginning your strength training routine or are a novice, we recommend strength training 20 to 30 minutes two to three days a week. If you're an old pro, you're most likely strength training 30 to 60 minutes four to five days a week, so keep it up!

 People over 60 who want to reduce their risk of falls and injury should start by strengthening legs, arms, and core muscles with two to three days of weight training a week for three to four weeks before walking long distances or engaging in aerobic exercise.

✔ **Flexibility training:** To maintain good muscle health and reduce injury, we urge you to incorporate flexibility training through stretching, yoga, and Pilates. These activities not only feel good but also increase the range of motion of your joints.

 Aerobic exercise with weight training using lighter weights and more repetitions is better than weight training alone using heavy, bulking-type weights and exercises.

In order for your routine to work and be effective, it has to be something you want to do and take full responsibility for. So, while you decide what kind of workout you want (weight training and aerobics), where you're going to get it (at the gym or on the bike trail), and which days of the week to devote to which activity (Monday: gym, Wednesday: rollerblade in the park, Thursday: swimming), personalize and work with your routine until it's comfortable.

If you haven't had much experience in the gym, start with some basic training. Many fitness centers offer circuit training, which consists of multiple machines with instructions and displays of the muscle groups that they target. You cycle through the machines, targeting all the muscle groups. You can increase the intensity as you go and concentrate on specific weak areas as you see fit. Aerobic activity can be worked into the schedule or you can alternate days between aerobic and strength training.

Getting the goods

You don't need to purchase expensive gym equipment to get a good workout. Here's a list of some basic equipment to get you started:

- ✔ **Handheld weights:** Hand weights (also known as *dumbbells*) are a must-have for any do-it-yourselfer. The most popular variety is vinyl-coated for comfort and easy grip and color-coded by weight. They range in increments from 1 to 10 pounds, and then go up to 12 and 15 pounds.

- ✔ **Resistance bands:** These bands are easy to use at any age or fitness level and offer your muscles a full-range-of-motion workout. Resistance bands are long tubes that look like rubber jump ropes with handles.

- ✔ **Exercise stability balls:** These balls offer numerous exercises and activities that activate and strengthen those hard-to-reach core muscles often overlooked during normal training. The balls come in a variety of sizes according to your height.

- ✔ **Floor mat:** A *closed-cell* (nonabsorbent to wick away moisture) foam mat that's at least ⅜ of an inch thick is great to avoid slipping, and to provide comfort and support.

✔ **Workout DVD:** You can find an endless variety of workouts for every age, lifestyle, and fitness level. Try one from your local movie rental store or your public library before you buy it.

✔ **Good quality shoes:** A comfortable and supportive pair of sneakers is essential. Make sure that your shoes have rubber soles and good arch support. More than anything, they should be comfortable.

Evaluating the success of your efforts

Sometimes, despite their best efforts, people encounter the slump of discouragement and frustration, especially when they've tried to lose weight more than once, only to gain it back. To bounce back from those self-defeating thoughts and feelings, refocus with the following methods:

✔ Focus on the process instead of the end result.

✔ Focus on what went well today (or this week) and the successes.

✔ Use visualization and imagery techniques to focus on yourself at your goal weight, participating in an enjoyable activity.

✔ Focus on physical activity as an opportunity to do something enjoyable.

✔ Put away the scale for awhile and focus on making lasting lifestyle changes. As a result, the weight will come off.

Finding the rewards at the end of your rainbow of sacrifices is easy. Every time you reach one of your goals, reward yourself. Every positive action deserves a pat on the back. Get some new clothes or take a mini-trip. And make sure that you set reasonable goals, because the rewards are that much more valuable.

A Microscopic Look at the Aging Brain

Keeping your brain function intact is probably high on your list of things to do as you age. Age can affect the complicated system of hormones, neurotransmitters, and nerves. In fact, the changes that can occur in the brain can be much more debilitating than some of the physical aspects of aging such as muscle and bone loss. In the next section, we look at exactly what happens to your brain as you age.

Normal physical changes

The ability to study the brain used to be limited to autopsies, but new brain imaging techniques have led to increased observation of age-related effects on the brain's structure and appearance.

The brain shrinks, the white matter thins, and the vital messengers in the brain diminish. Sounds scary, doesn't it? But relax! In most instances, you can compensate for age-related brain changes. You can expect the following as your brain ages:

✔ The brain's weight and volume decrease.

On average, the brain loses 10 percent of its weight, starting after the age of 20 with the abundance of loss coming after the age of 60.

- The *sulci* (grooves) on the surface of the brain widen.

- The brain starts to generate fewer messengers (the neurotransmitters).

- The brain can get accumulations of abnormal brain fibers made of protein, which are called *neurofibrillary tangles.* These plaques can cause Alzheimer's symptoms and are thought to contribute to age-related memory deficits.

- The accumulation of deposits of amyloid, an insoluble fibrous protein, in the brain cells is called *senile plaques.* Research is still not conclusive as to whether these plaques are part of normal aging.

How physical changes manifest through your mentality

One of the biggest fears people have of aging is losing their ability to think and remember. In regards to aging and the mind/body connection, a few categories of people exist:

- People who have a strong healthy body but are losing their minds

- Folks who are sharp as a tack with a deteriorating body

- The strong-bodied and strong-minded

The good news is that most people will be able to keep their cognitive faculties as they age unless they develop Alzheimer's or some other disease.

Changes in mental function that are part of normal aging

 Despite common belief, your memory doesn't worsen as you age. Memory does, however, change with age and these changes don't necessarily mean deterioration. In fact, memory becomes more accurate with age; you're just a bit slower at the processing part.

The most common normal change associated with aging is the ability to retrieve newly acquired information. In other words, your long-term memories remain intact, where as your short-term memory slows down.

So, when do all of these brain aging and short-term memory glitches start to occur? About 60 percent of people age 50 and older notice greater difficulty remembering names, dates, and other specific details. Memories associated with a specific time and place are most commonly effected. Thankfully, these small memory lapses — which are called *brain farts* as young adults or *senior moments* as you get older — aren't usually signs of a neurological disorder, such as Alzheimer's disease, but instead the result of normal changes in the structure and function of your brain.

Changes in mental function that may signify a health concern

Aging alone isn't the only cause of mental changes. Depression, dementia, side effects of drugs and alcohol, strokes, and head injury also cause mental changes, but these diseases aren't a universal occurrence. This leads us to the question, if some mental change is normal as you age, when should you be concerned and seek medical advice?

Don't panic. Ask yourself (or someone else, if you're not able to assess for yourself) if you're having any of the following changes in behavior or thinking processes. If you notice one or more of these signs in yourself or a loved one, or if someone tells you they've noticed these behaviors in you, see your healthcare professional for a full evaluation:

- ✔ Forgetting things more frequently than you used to (especially if a friend or family member tells you).

- ✔ Forgetting how to do familiar tasks.

- ✔ Difficulty learning new tasks.

- ✔ Being told that you told the same story within the same visit.

- ✔ Difficulty managing money, medications, and bills.

- ✔ Changes in personality such as anger or avoidance.

- ✔ Decreased hygiene.

There are other causes of abnormal mental function besides brain disease. Infections, medications, and other diseases can cause similar symptoms, so make sure that you or a loved one is evaluated by a doctor to get an accurate diagnosis if symptoms appear suddenly or seem to become worse.

Keeping Your Brain Young

So, you want to be as young as you *think?* There are certain steps you can take to keep the cobwebs in your mind at bay as you get older. In this section, we provide you with ways to keep your brain power strong.

Preventing age-related memory loss

The brain changes that come with age are inevitable — but they don't have to slow you down or trip you up. There are some medical, natural, and nutritional ways to increase and balance neurotransmitters when they do get out of balance.

 Be sure to consult with your healthcare provider before taking any medications, supplements, or beginning any other therapies for treating any perceived neurotransmitter deficiencies.

Check out these ways of staying alert and preventing memory loss:

✔ **Exercising your mind:** Mental stimulation and exercises can actually protect against cognitive losses. Most severe mental decline is from the disease processes instead of normal age-related function loss because as you age, the brain is able to make new connections if it's challenged and taken care of. Here are a few ways that you can challenge yourself:

- Play a musical instrument.

- Do crossword puzzles or other challenging board games.

- Socialize with family and friends.

- Start a new hobby.

- Stay interested and up-to-date on current events.

✔ **Staying physically active:** Regular exercise can improve blood flow to the brain. Exercise increases your metabolism and energy levels, which can help improve your attention span. If you exercise for as little as 30 to 45 minutes three times a week, studies show that you can improve age-related declines in your cognitive abilities.

✔ **Eating brain foods:** Neurotransmitter health requires the same balanced diet as the rest of your body — protein, carbohydrates, and fats. Three neurotransmitters are especially important to keep your brain functioning well:

- **Acetylcholine:** Foods rich in this chemical include egg yolks, peanuts, wheat germ, liver, meat, fish, milk, cheese, broccoli, cabbage, and cauliflower.

- **Dopamine:** These foods include all proteins, such as meat, milk products, fish, beans, nuts, and soy products.

- **Serotonin:** Serotonin-rich foods are carbohydrate-based, such as pasta, starchy vegetables, potatoes, cereals, and breads.

- **Drink plenty of water.** The brain is comprised of more water than any other organ in the body, at about 90 percent. Staying hydrated is essential for concentration and mental alertness, but how much water is enough? A good rule of thumb is to drink half of your body weight in ounces of water. If you drink coffee or alcohol, you have to add those ounces onto the total.

✔ **Drinking alcohol only in moderation:** People who drink heavily for years are at a higher risk of developing memory problems and dementia. We don't recommend drinking more than one to two drinks per day for men and one or less per day for women.

✔ **Stopping smoking:** Smoking is associated with dementia and one Dutch study found that smokers had twice the risk of developing Alzheimer's compared to those who never smoked. Smoking also has an increased risk of strokes, the other common type of dementia (multi-infarct).

✔ **Managing your stress:** Stress can cause the release of enzymes and hormones that can effect judgment and memory. Protein kinase C, cortisol, and corticosterone are a few that are thought to have a memory-impairing effect. These hormones are released in the body under normal stress situations, but it's not until they hang around too long as a result of chronic stressors that they affect memory.

✔ **Getting enough rest:** New evidence suggests that a regular pattern of eight hours of sleep per night helps protect you against age-related memory loss. Sleep experts say that having a regular sleep routine can improve cognition. Several studies discuss the similarities of sleep deprivation and age-related memory loss, but they're still researching the long-term effects of poor sleep and memory loss.

Improving Your Memory

What you consider a poor memory may just be less-than-effective habits when it comes to taking in and processing information. Barring disease, disorder, or injury, you can improve your ability to discover and retain information.

What type of memory are you losing?

Memory loss with normal aging results from the subtly changing environment within the brain. It's not clear exactly how much is actual memory loss and how much is the inability to quickly process the request for the information.

To help explain the differences between age-related memory loss and memory loss associated with brain disease, we discuss the different types of memory below:

- ✔ **Declarative:** This refers to memory that's consciously available. It's the type of memory that stores facts such as names, places, and times. Declarative memory is also referred to as conscious or cognitive memory and what most people refer to when they're experiencing lapses in their memory function.

- ✔ **Nondeclarative or procedural:** This type of memory relates to skills and routines. It consists of memory associated with motor learning, habits, perception, intuition, and conditioning. This area isn't affected much by aging.

- ✔ **Sensory:** This type of memory involves retaining something you have just seen or heard. It gives you the ability to see something for just a second and memorize it. Sensory memory isn't affected by aging as much as the other types of memory.

✔ **Short-term:** Short-term memory allows you to recall something from several seconds to as long as a minute without repetition. This area can be significantly affected by aging. This type is also one that can be improved with memory games and brain exercises.

✔ **Long-term:** Long-term memory can store much larger quantities of information for potentially unlimited duration — sometimes a whole lifetime. This area is little affected by normal aging.

Try putting some new information in your brain "next to" something you know you won't forget so you can retrieve it more easily. For example, if you meet someone new and want to remember his name is Robert, think of someone from your past or a childhood friend named Robert and create an association, then lock it down in your memory.

Figuring out how to remember

A good percentage of aging adults develop age-related memory loss, while some end up with the more aggressive memory deficits seen in diseases like Alzheimer's. Learning tools to help increase your ability to remember and recall, however, can help you retain as much of your thinking ability as possible. The following hints may help you remember important information:

✔ **Create memorable mental pictures and notes:** You remember things more easily if you can visualize them. If you're reading something and you read it out loud, you may retain it easier. Try to relate substance to items, such as colors, emotions, and textures, which can make more of an imprint in the brain.

✔ **Group things:** Group any new information to already stored info because it's easier to remember the group.

✔ **Organize:** Place objects such as keys in the same place. Use calendars for events and recurring occasions. Take notes, especially on complex material, and add pictures and colors to the notes to increase recall.

✔ **Repeat learned items:** The more times you repeat things or say them, the better the memory. After you meet someone, repeating the name out loud increases your ability to retain.

Want more? Go to dummies.com to receive 20% off on any Dummies title

Use promotion code DMTAR at checkout.

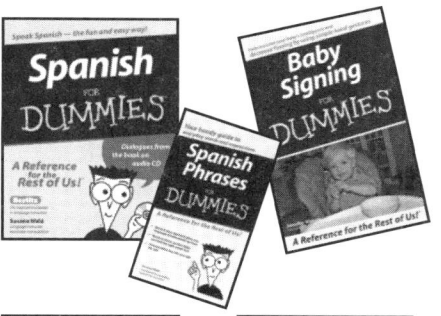
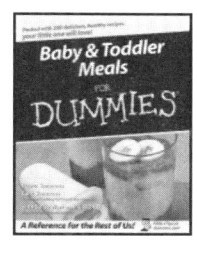
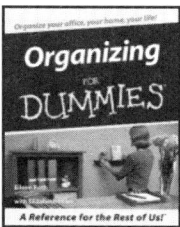
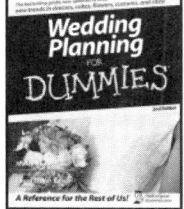
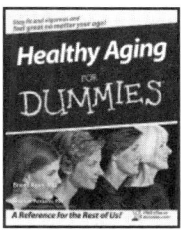
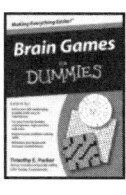
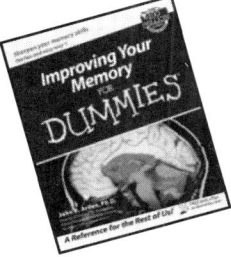
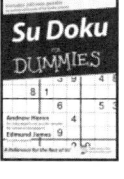

 Look for these titles wherever books are sold, call 877-762-2974, or visit dummies.com

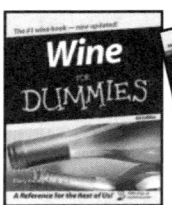 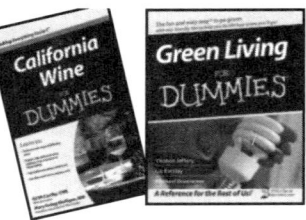 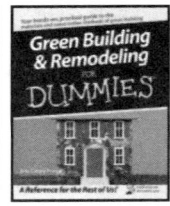

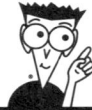 **With more than 1,400 titles to choose from, we've got a Dummies book for wherever you are in life!**

Business/Personal Finance & Investment

High-Powered Investing All-in-One For Dummies	9780470186268	$29.99
Investing For Dummies, 5th Edition	9780470289655	$21.99
Living Well in a Down Economy For Dummies	9780470401170	$14.99
Managing Your Money All-in-One For Dummies	9780470345467	$29.99
Personal Finance Workbook For Dummies	9780470099339	$19.99
Taxes 2009 For Dummies (January 2009)	9780470249512	$17.99

Crafts & Hobbies

California Wine For Dummies (May 2009)	9780470376072	$16.99
Canning & Preserving For Dummies	9780764524714	$16.99
Jewelry & Beading Designs For Dummies	9780470291122	$19.99
Knitting For Dummies, 2nd Edition	9780470287477	$21.99
Quilting For Dummies, 2nd Edition	9780764597992	$21.99
Watercolor Painting For Dummies	9780470182314	$24.99

Fitness & Diet

Dieting For Dummies, 2nd Edition	9780764541490	$21.99
Low-Calorie Dieting For Dummies	9780764599057	$21.99
Nutrition For Dummies, 4th Edition	9780471798682	$21.99
Exercise Balls For Dummies	9780764556234	$21.99
Fitness For Dummies, 3rd Edition	9780764578519	$21.99
Stretching For Dummies	9780470067413	$16.99

Want more? Go to dummies.com to receive 20% off on any Dummies title

Use promotion code DMTAR at checkout.

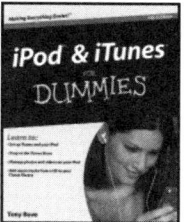

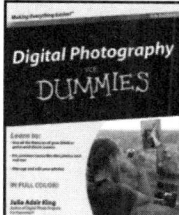

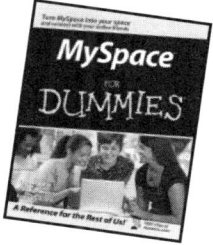

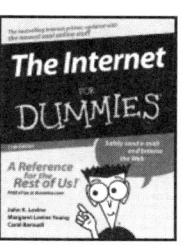

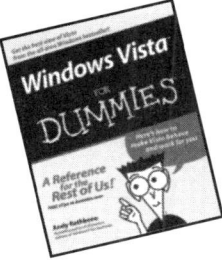

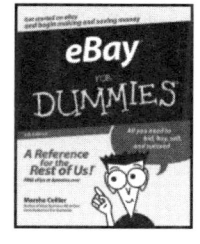

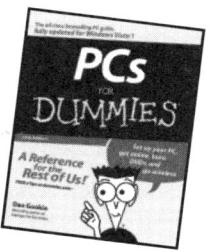

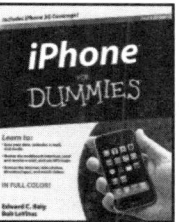

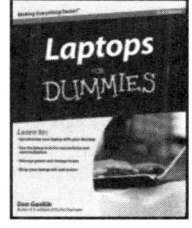

**Look for these titles wherever books are sold,
call 877-762-2974, or visit dummies.com**

Want more? Go to dummies.com to receive 20% off on any Dummies title
Use promotion code DMTAR at checkout.

Home & Business Computer Basics

Managing Your Life with Outlook For Dummies	9780471959304	$24.99
Excel 2007 All-in-One Desk Reference For Dummies	9780470037386	$29.99
Office 2007 All-in-One Desk Reference For Dummies	9780471782797	$29.99
BlackBerry For Dummies, 2nd Edition	9780470180792	$24.99
Computers For Seniors For Dummies	9780470240557	$19.99
iMac For Dummies, 5th Edition	9780470133866	$21.99
Macbook For Dummies, 2nd Edition	9780470278161	$24.99
PCs All-in-One Desk Reference For Dummies, 4th Edition	9780470223383	$29.99

Digital Life & Gadgets

CD & DVD Recording For Dummies, 2nd Edition	9780764559563	$21.99
Composing Digital Music For Dummies	9780470170953	$24.99
HDTV For Dummies, 2nd Edition	9780470096734	$21.99
Home Networking For Dummies, 4th Edition	9780470118061	$21.99
iPhone For Dummies, 2nd Edition	9780470423424	$21.99
Wii For Dummies	9780470173626	$21.99

Internet & Digital Media

Digital Photo Projects For Dummies	9780470121016	$34.99
Digital Photography For Dummies, 6th Edition	9780470250747	$24.99
Digital Video For Dummies, 4th Edition	9780471782780	$24.99
Shooting & Sharing Digital Photos For Dummies	9780764543593	$16.99
Blogging For Dummies, 2nd Edition	9780470230176	$21.99
eBay For Dummies, 5th Edition	9780470045299	$21.99
Facebook For Dummies	9780470262733	$21.99
Genealogy Online For Dummies, 5th Edition	9780470240571	$24.99
MySpace For Dummies, 2nd Edition	9780470275559	$21.99
YouTube For Dummies	9780470149256	$21.99

 Look for these titles wherever books are sold, call 877-762-2974, or visit dummies.com